Reversing Thr(

The Raw Vegan Plant-Based Detoxification & Regeneration Workbook for Healing Patients.

Volume 3

Health Central

Copyright © 2019

All rights reserved. Without limiting rights under the copyright reserved above, no part of this publication may be reproduced, stored, introduced into a retrieval system, distributed or transmitted in any form or by any means, including without limitation photocopying, recording, or other electronic or mechanical methods, without the prior written permission of the publisher, except in the case of brief quotations embodied in critical reviews and certain other non-commercial uses permitted by copyright law.

This book, with the opinions, suggestions and references made within it, is based on the author's personal experience and is for personal study and research purposes only. This program is about health and vitality, not disease. The author makes no medical claims. If you choose to use the material in this book on yourself, the author and publisher take no responsibility for your actions and decisions or the consequences thereof..

The scanning, uploading, and/or distribution of this document via the internet or via any other means without the permission of the publisher is illegal and is punishable by law. Please purchase only authorized editions and do not participate in or encourage electronic piracy of copyrightable materials

Quick recap of the healing protocol discussed in Volume 2:

1 – Take an Iris Diagnosis/Iridology session to identify all pre-existing conditions/weaknesses so these can be supported ASAP.

2 – Start sleeping at 10pm every night, and awaken when content.

3 – Introduce intermittent dry fasting into your routine (start off by simply delaying breakfast – and work from there – always listening to your body)

4 – Eat a diet of ONLY water dense fruits that we have tried and tested to work (grapes, oranges, melons, berries, mangos, etc) – sticking with a single type of fruit per meal, or per day.

5 – For maximum results, juice your fruit/vegetables.

6 – Throughout this protocol, for support, we recommend taking specific organ glandulars and herbs for weaker organs/pre-existing weaknesses (the kidneys almost always need supporting as they offload your body's toxic load)

7 – Do it with others and spread this powerful knowledge to those you love.

Cravings! Oh Cravings...

So life is wonderful and full of vitality. Your consciousness has increased and your body's biology is balancing out as you live as a Fruigivore. Having experienced and accepted that we as human beings thrive on fruit, you are starting to see the benefits.

However, there are still times that you have powerful cravings for cooked foods such as pizza, fries, potato chips, burgers, etc. Where are these cravings randomly coming from? Why do they come on so strongly? How can you overcome these cravings?

As the fruit disposes of the parasites, they put up a fight because they do not want to leave – they need feeding and NOW! This manifests itself through strong cravings that can feel very challenging to overcome.

Parasites dislike energy and Oxygen, therefore they thrive on foods that have zero electromagnetic energy, with their favourites being cooked fats, starches, dairy and meat products. Fruit is nourishing life-giving food which comes with an un-matched detoxifying power and it is loaded with energy. Parasites struggle to adapt to a fruit diet hence why they trigger cravings.

Throughout our work, Fructose (fruit sugar) has worked well in the removal of parasites from the body. The addition of herbs can support this but in general, fruit alone is highly capable of performing well.
You should see results within two to three weeks. Cravings will strike within this period - just remind yourself that this is a sign of the parasites passing away. As you alkalize and hydrate your body, the parasites will be struggling to survive so be sure to push through these feelings and keep moving forward with your protocol.

Parasites struggle to stay alive also with a diet rich in leafy green vegetables because they contain chlorophyll and this is full of electricity and Oxygen. However, fruit is far more hydrating and therefore much more effective.

If you are finding that your cravings are unbearable – then it would be wise to get yourself onto a parasite removal herbal formula. We have had good feedback from this kit: **CureMyParasite.com**

Remove social triggers and situations that increase your desire for cooked/low energy foods. For example, many patients have found that they previously found themselves eating cooked foods more so during events, or friends/family gatherings. Be mindful of this and perhaps have a fruit salad prepared beforehand. You could also work towards showing your circle of friends and family the benefits that this protocol brings so they could also potentially join you. Getting yourself an accountability partner works well too.

Another very useful technique to become more mindful and present is to meditate. We teach a variety of meditation methods to clients that are struggling to overcome strong craving attacks. A simple routine would be to calm your breathing down, relax, and focus on imagining a healing and soothing light enter into your body through your head – feel it nourish and untangle any blocked energy or resistance within that is causing these cravings to want to take over. Let this glowing light channel out all negative and non-productive thoughts and feelings – far out of your body through your finger tips and toes – with every breath you breath out, feel these craving feelings leave your body. This is one tried and tested routine that we have found to work – give it a try and feel the presence and calmness within.

Once you get through the early stages of your fruitarian diet, the chemistry within your body will start to change and you will begin noticing that you are more attracted to the beautiful and differing colours of fruits (and vegetables). Your consciousness will increase towards nature and fellow humans.

Fruits will elevate your consciousness to a higher state whilst cooked foods will numb and suppress your progress. A fruit-based diet will make you face your daily challenges head on and work through them, as opposed to cooked foods which will drain you of energy, contribute towards a slower mentality and make you put off tasks to another day. Cooked foods will contribute towards holding you back, and stop you from healing, and becoming stronger as a person, both mentally and physically.

The major positive is that fruit is generally available in abundance – you could even grow some yourself – it is very sustainable - and providing it has been picked ripe, you will get to experience the taste of true satisfying sweetness that will heal you whilst starving out and removing all unwanted parasites.

If you give into your cravings – you will set yourself back and if you continue to feed your parasites / fungus / worms – they will continue to live and breed within your body's environment. Just like human-beings, parasites defecate – but they don't have a bathroom, so your struggling body ends up being the victim of their waste matter. This leads to an increase in your toxic load and the creation of uric acid in the body. With yet more acids to contend with, your inflammation levels increase – leading to increased irritation and mental imbalances.

It is actually very easy to detoxify yourself. YOU CAN DO THIS – just stay strong and blast these creatures out of your system with fruit (and green juices).

Having eaten cooked foods for the majority of your lifetime, it can be challenging to move over to a pure fruit diet, and this is why we recommend a transition period which involves the allowance of steamed starch-free vegetables, dried fruit (dates, figs, mango, raisins), avocados, bananas, tasty salads, vegetable broth – for dinner. Providing you are eating fruit during the daytime, you can follow this regimen for as long as it takes you to move over to a 100% fruit diet. Ensure you load up on the fruit before dinner time, so you feel full and satisfied by the end of the day.

We recommend steamed vegetables and salads for dinner/evening time mainly because this is when the parasites tend to strike. They feed in the evenings because they prefer to come out during darkness instead of daylight. The majority of our patients have also reported cravings during the evening to night time periods.

Hunger is another important topic to address. If you are hungry – this is normally a sign that you are not eating enough fruit / not consuming sufficient calories. With fruit being much lower in calories, you have to eat much more of it in order to reach your individual caloric requirement. A couple of pieces will not suffice – you will need several pieces in order to feel satiated and carry yourself over to your next meal time.

In the early stages, you should over-indulge during your fruit meal times and as you improve, you can adjust this accordingly. You have nothing to be worried about when over-consuming fruit because it is the food intended for our species and it is designed specifically for our bodies to digest easily. The added benefit is that fruit / fructose (fruit sugar) is alive and alkaline unlike processed sugar which is acid-forming to the body.

If your body is struggling to process fructose, this will likely point towards an issue within specific organs but once these have been cleansed and the toxic acids within your body have moved out, you will thrive on fruits. As soon as you adjust to the fruits that were intended for you by nature, eating mucus-forming / cooked starchy foods will just leave you with extreme fatigue because your body will struggle to process and digest these low energy foods that were never meant for it. You will become sensitive to acid-forming foods and your body's reaction to them will tell you everything you need to know.

Note: We have found cravings to also be a result of emotional imbalances and "comfort eating". If you have weak adrenal glands, then you may suffer from this. In this case, we would need to focus on un-clogging your adrenal glands (and all related pathways/organs) through herbs, fasting and fruit – and transitioning you gently into a longer-term detoxification protocol.

Are you ready to become enlightened and move to a higher state of consciousness whilst reversing your conditions? Do you want to be free of anxiety, prolonged sadness and depression? Gift yourself with vibrant health and spiritual evolution – get back to nature and connect with the foods that were made for us to thrive on.

Our goal throughout this workbook is to help you with recording your progress and applying the information stated in this section.

Start with what you are most comfortable with and make it enjoyable, choose your favourite sweet fruits. If you deviate from the routine, we advise to get back on track as soon as possible. Just keep moving forward, keep track of progress, and be persistent.

We would like to wish you all the best and if you would like to book a consultation, or if you have any questions, thoughts, or comments, feel free to email us at:

HealingCentral8@gmail.com

Good Luck with your healing journey.

Tried & Tested Fruit Juicer: **YourFruitJuicer.com**

Tried & Tested Vegetable Juicer: **YourVegJuicer.com**

Unwanted Meaty/Starchy/Cheesy Food Cravings?

CureMyParasite.com

[EXAMPLE 1]
Today's Date: 2nd Jan 2019

Morning
I just ate 3 mangoes - very sweet and tasty. I felt a heavy feeling under my chest area so I stopped eating. Unsure what that was - maybe digestive or the transverse colon?

Afternoon
I was feeling hungry so I am eating some dried figs, pineapple and apricots with around 750ml of spring water.

Evening
Sipping on a green tea (herbal). Feeling pretty strong and alert at the moment.

Night
Enjoying a bowl of red seeded grapes. Currently I feel satisfied.

Today's Notes (Highlights, Thoughts, Feelings):

Unlike yesterday, today was a good day. I am noticing an increase in regular bowel movements which makes me feel cleansed and light afterwards. I feel as though my kidneys are also starting to filter better (white sediment visible in morning wee).

It definitely helps to document my thoughts in this workbook. A great way to reflect, improve and stay on track.

Feeling very good - vibrant and strong - I have noticed a major improvement in my physical fitness and performance. Mentally I feel healthier and happier.

[EXAMPLE 2]
Today's Date: 3rd Jan 2019

Morning
Dry fasting (water and food free since 8pm last night) - will go up until 12:30pm today, and start with 500ml of spring water before eating half a watermelon.

Afternoon
Kept busy and was in and out quite a bit - so nothing consumed.

Evening
At around 5pm, I had a peppermint tea with a selection of mixed dried fruit (small bowl of apricot, dates, mango, pineapple, and prunes).

Night
Sipped on spring water through the evening as required.
Finished off the other half of the watermelon from the morning.

Today's Notes (Highlights, Thoughts, Feelings):

As with most days, today started well with me dry fasting (continuing my fast from my sleep/skipping breakfast) up until around 12:30pm and then eating half a watermelon. The laxative effect of the watermelon helped me poop and release any loosened toxins from the fasting period.
I tend to struggle on some days from 3pm onwards. Up until that point I am okay but if the cravings strike then it can be challenging. I remind myself that those burgers and chips do not have any live healing energy.
I feel good in general. I feel fantastic doing a fruit/juice fast but slightly empty by the end of the day.
Cooked food makes me feel severe fatigue and mental fog.
Will continue with my fruit fasting and start to introduce fruit juices due to their deeper detox benefits. I would love to be on juices only as I have seen others within the community achieve amazing results.

[EXAMPLE 3]
Today's Date: 4th Jan 2019

Morning
Today I woke and my children were enjoying some watermelon for breakfast - and the smell was luring so I joined them. Large bowl of watermelon eaten at around 8am. Started with a glass of water.

Afternoon
Snacked on left over watermelon throughout the morning and afternoon. Had 5 dates an hour or so after.

Evening
Had around 3 mangoes at around 6pm. Felt content - but then I was invited round to a family gathering where a selection of pizzas, burgers and chips were being served. I gave into the peer pressure and felt like I let myself down!

Night
Having over-eaten earlier on in the evening, I was still feeling bloated with a headache (possibly digestion related) and I also felt quite mucus filled (wheez in chest and coughing up phlegm). Very sleepy and low energy. The perils of cooked foods!!

Today's Notes (Highlights, Thoughts, Feelings):

I let myself down today. It all started well until I ate a fully blown meal (and over-ate). I didn't remain focussed and I spun off track. As a result my energy levels were much lower and I felt a bout of extreme fatigue 30 minutes after the meal (most likely the body struggling to with digesting all that cooked food).
I need to stick to the plan because the difference between fruit fasting, and eating cooked foods is huge - 1 makes you feel empowered whilst the other makes you feel drained. I also felt the mucus overload after the meal - it kicked in pretty quickly.
Today I felt disappointed after giving in to the meal but tomorrow is a new day and I will keep on going! It is important to remind myself that I won't get better if I cannot stick to the routine.

Frequently Asked Questions

Can I spray vitamin B12 (and other vitamins/minerals/supplements) onto my fruit?

Yes, if you are heavily deficient in the initial stages. Within the broad range of fruits available today, you will find all nutrients present (all biologically available and easily absorbed by the body). This raw diet is far superior to anything else out there as it was originally intended for the human body. If you initially have deficiencies then you may opt to use supplementation but with time, as your body normalises/detoxifies and adapts, you will find that you will no longer be deficient in anything, and your absorption of nutrients from food will also return (all of our patients initially suffer from mal-absorption due to congestion in the gut).

It is hard for me to dry fast as I get thirsty regularly. Is it okay for me to do a water fast?

Water fasting works well and you will find great benefit in this. You could even slow juice your fruit (and some vegetables if needed) and perform a fast purely on juiced fruit - this would be more powerful. Many within the Fruitarian community talk about this and the "solid food vacation". Do try to work your way up to dry fasting (hint: you dry fast during sleep). Be sure to support your kidneys and adrenal glands with either herbs or kidney and adrenal glandular capsules because the toxic load leaving your body via your skin, and kidneys will be highly concentrated in acidity and could knock them harshly - so be aware of this.

How am I supposed to stay full on an all-fruit diet?

We don't recommend just jumping straight into an all-fruit diet immediately. During the transition stages of moving from cooked foods to a fruit diet, we recommend that you increase your fruit intake each time you feel hungry and in addition make a large salad to serve as a filler. The salad could consist of lettuce, any leafy greens, tomatoes, cucumber, onions, sweet-corn, mushrooms, avocado (mashed up as the sauce), lemon juice, and even some optional tahini (crushed sesame seed paste). This is just one sample recipe – there are many ways to make a delicious salad. Many choose to also make a variety of raw zucchini spaghetti dishes with the sauce being made of blended tomatoes, sun-dried tomatoes, basil, onions and a dash of garlic. Again, this is just one example – with research, you will discover many more tasty recipes that can really support you in the transition phase. Always aim to return to fruit – this should be your default diet.

Today's Date:

Morning
(work towards continuing your night time dry fast up until at least 12pm)

Afternoon
(get hydrating with fresh fruit or even better slow juiced fruits/berries/melons)

Evening
(aim to wind down to a dry fast by around 6pm to 7pm)

Night
(work your way up to dry fasting from the evening until 12pm the following day)

Today's Notes (Highlights, Thoughts, Feelings, What Could You Improve On?)

"Get yourself an accountability partner to complete a 3 month detox with. Start with 7 days and work your way up. It will be fun and motivating completing it with somebody (or a group) ...or of course you can go it alone"

Today's Date:

——————————— Morning ———————————
(work towards continuing your night time dry fast up until at least 12pm)

——————————— Afternoon ———————————
(get hydrating with fresh fruit or even better slow juiced fruits/berries/melons)

——————————— Evening ———————————
(aim to wind down to a dry fast by around 6pm to 7pm)

——————————— Night ———————————
(work your way up to dry fasting from the evening until 12pm the following day)

Today's Notes (Highlights, Thoughts, Feelings, What Could You Improve On?)

"Remember to keep yourself hydrated with water too (spring water preferred)."

_____
Today's Date:
_____ **Morning** _____
(work towards continuing your night time dry fast up until at least 12pm)

_____ **Afternoon** _____
(get hydrating with fresh fruit or even better slow juiced fruits/berries/melons)

_____ **Evening** _____
(aim to wind down to a dry fast by around 6pm to 7pm)

_____ **Night** _____
(work your way up to dry fasting from the evening until 12pm the following day)

_____

Today's Notes (Highlights, Thoughts, Feelings, What Could You Improve On?)

"Eat melons/watermelons separately, and before any other fruit as it digests faster and we want to limit fermentation (acidity) which can occur if other fruits are mixed in."

Today's Date:

———————————— **Morning** ————————————
(work towards continuing your night time dry fast up until at least 12pm)

———————————— **Afternoon** ————————————
(get hydrating with fresh fruit or even better slow juiced fruits/berries/melons)

———————————— **Evening** ————————————
(aim to wind down to a dry fast by around 6pm to 7pm)

———————————— **Night** ————————————
(work your way up to dry fasting from the evening until 12pm the following day)

Today's Notes (Highlights, Thoughts, Feelings, What Could You Improve On?)

"Stay focussed on the end goal of removing mucus & toxins from your body and feeling wonderful again!"

Today's Date:

Morning
(work towards continuing your night time dry fast up until at least 12pm)

Afternoon
(get hydrating with fresh fruit or even better slow juiced fruits/berries/melons)

Evening
(aim to wind down to a dry fast by around 6pm to 7pm)

Night
(work your way up to dry fasting from the evening until 12pm the following day)

Today's Notes (Highlights, Thoughts, Feelings, What Could You Improve On?)

"Meditate and perform deep breathing exercises in order to help yourself remain present minded and stay on track."

Today's Date:

―――――――――――― **Morning** ――――――――――――
(work towards continuing your night time dry fast up until at least 12pm)

―――――――――――― **Afternoon** ――――――――――――
(get hydrating with fresh fruit or even better slow juiced fruits/berries/melons)

―――――――――――― **Evening** ――――――――――――
(aim to wind down to a dry fast by around 6pm to 7pm)

―――――――――――― **Night** ――――――――――――
(work your way up to dry fasting from the evening until 12pm the following day)

Today's Notes (Highlights, Thoughts, Feelings, What Could You Improve On?)

"Join a few like-minded communities – there are many juicing and raw vegan based groups, both online and offline. Being part of a community can help motivate you to reach your goals."

Today's Date:

─────────── **Morning** ───────────
(work towards continuing your night time dry fast up until at least 12pm)

─────────── **Afternoon** ───────────
(get hydrating with fresh fruit or even better slow juiced fruits/berries/melons)

─────────── **Evening** ───────────
(aim to wind down to a dry fast by around 6pm to 7pm)

─────────── **Night** ───────────
(work your way up to dry fasting from the evening until 12pm the following day)

Today's Notes (Highlights, Thoughts, Feelings, What Could You Improve On?)

"If you are struggling with hunger pangs in the early stages, try some dates or dried apricots, prunes, or raisins, with a cup of herbal tea.

Today's Date:

─────────────── **Morning** ───────────────
(work towards continuing your night time dry fast up until at least 12pm)

─────────────── **Afternoon** ───────────────
(get hydrating with fresh fruit or even better slow juiced fruits/berries/melons)

─────────────── **Evening** ───────────────
(aim to wind down to a dry fast by around 6pm to 7pm)

─────────────── **Night** ───────────────
(work your way up to dry fasting from the evening until 12pm the following day)

Today's Notes (Highlights, Thoughts, Feelings, What Could You Improve On?)

"Get into a routine of regularly buying fresh fruit (or grow your own if weather permits) to keep your supplies up."

Today's Date:

———————————— **Morning** ————————————
(work towards continuing your night time dry fast up until at least 12pm)

———————————— **Afternoon** ————————————
(get hydrating with fresh fruit or even better slow juiced fruits/berries/melons)

———————————— **Evening** ————————————
(aim to wind down to a dry fast by around 6pm to 7pm)

———————————— **Night** ————————————
(work your way up to dry fasting from the evening until 12pm the following day)

Today's Notes (Highlights, Thoughts, Feelings, What Could You Improve On?)

"Regularly remind yourself about the great rewards and benefits that you will experience from keeping up this detox."

Today's Date:

Morning
(work towards continuing your night time dry fast up until at least 12pm)

Afternoon
(get hydrating with fresh fruit or even better slow juiced fruits/berries/melons)

Evening
(aim to wind down to a dry fast by around 6pm to 7pm)

Night
(work your way up to dry fasting from the evening until 12pm the following day)

Today's Notes (Highlights, Thoughts, Feelings, What Could You Improve On?)

"Keep your teeth brushed and flossed regularly – at least twice a day to keep them healthy for your fruit sessions. You will notice an improvement in your dental health with this raw/fruit diet."

Today's Date:

———————————— **Morning** ————————————
(work towards continuing your night time dry fast up until at least 12pm)

———————————— **Afternoon** ————————————
(get hydrating with fresh fruit or even better slow juiced fruits/berries/melons)

———————————— **Evening** ————————————
(aim to wind down to a dry fast by around 6pm to 7pm)

———————————— **Night** ————————————
(work your way up to dry fasting from the evening until 12pm the following day)

Today's Notes (Highlights, Thoughts, Feelings, What Could You Improve On?)

"Be motivated by the vision of becoming an example for others to learn from and follow."

Today's Date:

--- **Morning** ---

(work towards continuing your night time dry fast up until at least 12pm)

--- **Afternoon** ---

(get hydrating with fresh fruit or even better slow juiced fruits/berries/melons)

--- **Evening** ---

(aim to wind down to a dry fast by around 6pm to 7pm)

--- **Night** ---

(work your way up to dry fasting from the evening until 12pm the following day)

Today's Notes (Highlights, Thoughts, Feelings, What Could You Improve On?)

"Embrace your achievements and wonderful results – feel and appreciate the difference within you as a result of this new routine."

Today's Date:

———————————— Morning ————————————

(work towards continuing your night time dry fast up until at least 12pm)

———————————— Afternoon ————————————

(get hydrating with fresh fruit or even better slow juiced fruits/berries/melons)

———————————— Evening ————————————

(aim to wind down to a dry fast by around 6pm to 7pm)

———————————— Night ————————————

(work your way up to dry fasting from the evening until 12pm the following day)

Today's Notes (Highlights, Thoughts, Feelings, What Could You Improve On?)

"Buy fruit in bulk where possible so you have ample supplies for a week or two in advance. If in a hot climate, you could even freeze your fruit or make ice lollies out of it (crush & freeze)."

Today's Date:

Morning
(work towards continuing your night time dry fast up until at least 12pm)

Afternoon
(get hydrating with fresh fruit or even better slow juiced fruits/berries/melons)

Evening
(aim to wind down to a dry fast by around 6pm to 7pm)

Night
(work your way up to dry fasting from the evening until 12pm the following day)

Today's Notes (Highlights, Thoughts, Feelings, What Could You Improve On?)

"Stay as busy as you can during the daytime. Creating a busy routine makes it easier to manage your diet."

Today's Date:

Morning
(work towards continuing your night time dry fast up until at least 12pm)

Afternoon
(get hydrating with fresh fruit or even better slow juiced fruits/berries/melons)

Evening
(aim to wind down to a dry fast by around 6pm to 7pm)

Night
(work your way up to dry fasting from the evening until 12pm the following day)

Today's Notes (Highlights, Thoughts, Feelings, What Could You Improve On?)

"Complete your fruit and fasting routine with a group of friends/family/colleagues so you can all support one another."

Today's Date:

———————————————— **Morning** ————————————————

(work towards continuing your night time dry fast up until at least 12pm)

———————————————— **Afternoon** ————————————————

(get hydrating with fresh fruit or even better slow juiced fruits/berries/melons)

———————————————— **Evening** ————————————————

(aim to wind down to a dry fast by around 6pm to 7pm)

———————————————— **Night** ————————————————

(work your way up to dry fasting from the evening until 12pm the following day)

Today's Notes (Highlights, Thoughts, Feelings, What Could You Improve On?)

"Monitor your urine regularly. Urinate in a jar and leave overnight. If you see a thick cloud of white sediment (success!), your kidneys are filtering acids out."

Today's Date:

———————————————— **Morning** ————————————————
(work towards continuing your night time dry fast up until at least 12pm)

———————————————— **Afternoon** ————————————————
(get hydrating with fresh fruit or even better slow juiced fruits/berries/melons)

———————————————— **Evening** ————————————————
(aim to wind down to a dry fast by around 6pm to 7pm)

———————————————— **Night** ————————————————
(work your way up to dry fasting from the evening until 12pm the following day)

Today's Notes (Highlights, Thoughts, Feelings, What Could You Improve On?)

"Have genuine love and care for yourself. If craving junk food, affirm positive inner talk ("if I eat this, I won't feel good so leave it out")."

Today's Date:

―――――――――――――― **Morning** ――――――――――――――

(work towards continuing your night time dry fast up until at least 12pm)

―――――――――――――― **Afternoon** ――――――――――――――

(get hydrating with fresh fruit or even better slow juiced fruits/berries/melons)

―――――――――――――― **Evening** ――――――――――――――

(aim to wind down to a dry fast by around 6pm to 7pm)

―――――――――――――― **Night** ――――――――――――――

(work your way up to dry fasting from the evening until 12pm the following day)

Today's Notes (Highlights, Thoughts, Feelings, What Could You Improve On?)

"Filter out unwanted acids with this alkaline water-dense fruits protocol."

Today's Date: _____

──────────────── **Morning** ────────────────

(work towards continuing your night time dry fast up until at least 12pm)

──────────────── **Afternoon** ────────────────

(get hydrating with fresh fruit or even better slow juiced fruits/berries/melons)

──────────────── **Evening** ────────────────

(aim to wind down to a dry fast by around 6pm to 7pm)

──────────────── **Night** ────────────────

(work your way up to dry fasting from the evening until 12pm the following day)

Today's Notes (Highlights, Thoughts, Feelings, What Could You Improve On?)

"Look out for white cloud/sediment (acids) in your urine to confirm kidney filtration."

Today's Date:

——————————— **Morning** ———————————

(work towards continuing your night time dry fast up until at least 12pm)

——————————— **Afternoon** ———————————

(get hydrating with fresh fruit or even better slow juiced fruits/berries/melons)

——————————— **Evening** ———————————

(aim to wind down to a dry fast by around 6pm to 7pm)

——————————— **Night** ———————————

(work your way up to dry fasting from the evening until 12pm the following day)

Today's Notes (Highlights, Thoughts, Feelings, What Could You Improve On?)

"Infections emerge in an acidic environment"

Today's Date:

──────────────── **Morning** ────────────────
(work towards continuing your night time dry fast up until at least 12pm)

──────────────── **Afternoon** ────────────────
(get hydrating with fresh fruit or even better slow juiced fruits/berries/melons)

──────────────── **Evening** ────────────────
(aim to wind down to a dry fast by around 6pm to 7pm)

──────────────── **Night** ────────────────
(work your way up to dry fasting from the evening until 12pm the following day)

Today's Notes (Highlights, Thoughts, Feelings, What Could You Improve On?)

"Any deficiencies that you may have will disappear once you have cleansed your clogged up gut/colon, kidneys and various other eliminative organs."

Today's Date:

Morning
(work towards continuing your night time dry fast up until at least 12pm)

Afternoon
(get hydrating with fresh fruit or even better slow juiced fruits/berries/melons)

Evening
(aim to wind down to a dry fast by around 6pm to 7pm)

Night
(work your way up to dry fasting from the evening until 12pm the following day)

Today's Notes (Highlights, Thoughts, Feelings, What Could You Improve On?)

"Dependant on how deeply you detox yourself, you could even eliminate any genetic weaknesses that you may have inherited."

Today's Date:

———————————— Morning ————————————
(work towards continuing your night time dry fast up until at least 12pm)

———————————— Afternoon ————————————
(get hydrating with fresh fruit or even better slow juiced fruits/berries/melons)

———————————— Evening ————————————
(aim to wind down to a dry fast by around 6pm to 7pm)

———————————— Night ————————————
(work your way up to dry fasting from the evening until 12pm the following day)

Today's Notes (Highlights, Thoughts, Feelings, What Could You Improve On?)

"Keep focused on your detox. Even past injuries / trauma are all repairable for good."

Today's Date:

_____ **Morning** _____

(work towards continuing your night time dry fast up until at least 12pm)

_____ **Afternoon** _____

(get hydrating with fresh fruit or even better slow juiced fruits/berries/melons)

_____ **Evening** _____

(aim to wind down to a dry fast by around 6pm to 7pm)

_____ **Night** _____

(work your way up to dry fasting from the evening until 12pm the following day)

Today's Notes (Highlights, Thoughts, Feelings, What Could You Improve On?)

"If you suffer from ongoing sadness / depression, a deep detox will support your mental health. You will soon notice a positive change in your mood."

Today's Date:

Morning
(work towards continuing your night time dry fast up until at least 12pm)

Afternoon
(get hydrating with fresh fruit or even better slow juiced fruits/berries/melons)

Evening
(aim to wind down to a dry fast by around 6pm to 7pm)

Night
(work your way up to dry fasting from the evening until 12pm the following day)

Today's Notes (Highlights, Thoughts, Feelings, What Could You Improve On?)

"Have your fruits/juices throughout the day. As the evening approaches, start to dry fast – your body wants to rest and heal from this point on."

Today's Date:

———————————— **Morning** ————————————
(work towards continuing your night time dry fast up until at least 12pm)

———————————— **Afternoon** ————————————
(get hydrating with fresh fruit or even better slow juiced fruits/berries/melons)

———————————— **Evening** ————————————
(aim to wind down to a dry fast by around 6pm to 7pm)

———————————— **Night** ————————————
(work your way up to dry fasting from the evening until 12pm the following day)

Today's Notes (Highlights, Thoughts, Feelings, What Could You Improve On?)

"The kidneys dislike proteins but really appreciate juicy fruits like melons, berries, citrus fruits, pineapples, mangoes, apples, grapes."

Today's Date:

―――――――――――――― **Morning** ――――――――――――――

(work towards continuing your night time dry fast up until at least 12pm)

―――――――――――――― **Afternoon** ――――――――――――――

(get hydrating with fresh fruit or even better slow juiced fruits/berries/melons)

―――――――――――――― **Evening** ――――――――――――――

(aim to wind down to a dry fast by around 6pm to 7pm)

―――――――――――――― **Night** ――――――――――――――

(work your way up to dry fasting from the evening until 12pm the following day)

Today's Notes (Highlights, Thoughts, Feelings, What Could You Improve On?)

"Healing is very easy. There's no need to complicate it. Keep it simple and you will see results."

Today's Date:

Morning
(work towards continuing your night time dry fast up until at least 12pm)

Afternoon
(get hydrating with fresh fruit or even better slow juiced fruits/berries/melons)

Evening
(aim to wind down to a dry fast by around 6pm to 7pm)

Night
(work your way up to dry fasting from the evening until 12pm the following day)

Today's Notes (Highlights, Thoughts, Feelings, What Could You Improve On?)

"Keep your body in an alkaline state as this is where regeneration takes place."

Today's Date:

Morning
(work towards continuing your night time dry fast up until at least 12pm)

Afternoon
(get hydrating with fresh fruit or even better slow juiced fruits/berries/melons)

Evening
(aim to wind down to a dry fast by around 6pm to 7pm)

Night
(work your way up to dry fasting from the evening until 12pm the following day)

Today's Notes (Highlights, Thoughts, Feelings, What Could You Improve On?)

"A daily enema with boiled water (cooled down) will support your detox greatly."

Today's Date:

Morning
(work towards continuing your night time dry fast up until at least 12pm)

Afternoon
(get hydrating with fresh fruit or even better slow juiced fruits/berries/melons)

Evening
(aim to wind down to a dry fast by around 6pm to 7pm)

Night
(work your way up to dry fasting from the evening until 12pm the following day)

Today's Notes (Highlights, Thoughts, Feelings, What Could You Improve On?)

"Have your iris' read by an iridologist that works with Dr Bernard Jensen's system."

Today's Date:

──────────────── **Morning** ────────────────

(work towards continuing your night time dry fast up until at least 12pm)

──────────────── **Afternoon** ────────────────

(get hydrating with fresh fruit or even better slow juiced fruits/berries/melons)

──────────────── **Evening** ────────────────

(aim to wind down to a dry fast by around 6pm to 7pm)

──────────────── **Night** ────────────────

(work your way up to dry fasting from the evening until 12pm the following day)

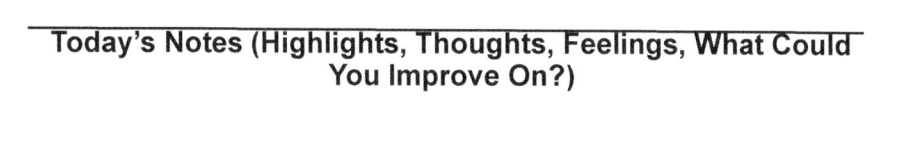

Today's Notes (Highlights, Thoughts, Feelings, What Could You Improve On?)

"Take a herbal parasite formula for a month. It will eliminate food cravings. This is an important point."

Today's Date:

──────────────── **Morning** ────────────────

(work towards continuing your night time dry fast up until at least 12pm)

──────────────── **Afternoon** ────────────────

(get hydrating with fresh fruit or even better slow juiced fruits/berries/melons)

──────────────── **Evening** ────────────────

(aim to wind down to a dry fast by around 6pm to 7pm)

──────────────── **Night** ────────────────

(work your way up to dry fasting from the evening until 12pm the following day)

Today's Notes (Highlights, Thoughts, Feelings, What Could You Improve On?)

"Your skin is the largest eliminative organ. Skin brushing and sweating are crucial. Sauna heat is ideal, steam can also work."

Today's Date:

———————————— **Morning** ————————————

(work towards continuing your night time dry fast up until at least 12pm)

———————————— **Afternoon** ————————————

(get hydrating with fresh fruit or even better slow juiced fruits/berries/melons)

———————————— **Evening** ————————————

(aim to wind down to a dry fast by around 6pm to 7pm)

———————————— **Night** ————————————

(work your way up to dry fasting from the evening until 12pm the following day)

Today's Notes (Highlights, Thoughts, Feelings, What Could You Improve On?)

"If you are on medications, monitor the relevant statistics (e.g. blood pressure, blood sugar level, etc). Upon improving, lower medication"

Today's Date:

Morning
(work towards continuing your night time dry fast up until at least 12pm)

Afternoon
(get hydrating with fresh fruit or even better slow juiced fruits/berries/melons)

Evening
(aim to wind down to a dry fast by around 6pm to 7pm)

Night
(work your way up to dry fasting from the evening until 12pm the following day)

Today's Notes (Highlights, Thoughts, Feelings, What Could You Improve On?)

"Most people do not breathe effectively. Your body requires a healthy supply of oxygen to heal. Practice breathing techniques daily."

Today's Date:

— **Morning** —

(work towards continuing your night time dry fast up until at least 12pm)

— **Afternoon** —

(get hydrating with fresh fruit or even better slow juiced fruits/berries/melons)

— **Evening** —

(aim to wind down to a dry fast by around 6pm to 7pm)

— **Night** —

(work your way up to dry fasting from the evening until 12pm the following day)

Today's Notes (Highlights, Thoughts, Feelings, What Could You Improve On?)

"Disease is not the presence of something evil, but rather the lack of the presence of something essential."
— Dr. Bernard Jensen.

Today's Date:

Morning
(work towards continuing your night time dry fast up until at least 12pm)

Afternoon
(get hydrating with fresh fruit or even better slow juiced fruits/berries/melons)

Evening
(aim to wind down to a dry fast by around 6pm to 7pm)

Night
(work your way up to dry fasting from the evening until 12pm the following day)

Today's Notes (Highlights, Thoughts, Feelings, What Could You Improve On?)

"Fruits will empower you, providing live energy. Cooked foods in comparison will use vital energy that could otherwise be used for healing."

Today's Date:

Morning
(work towards continuing your night time dry fast up until at least 12pm)

Afternoon
(get hydrating with fresh fruit or even better slow juiced fruits/berries/melons)

Evening
(aim to wind down to a dry fast by around 6pm to 7pm)

Night
(work your way up to dry fasting from the evening until 12pm the following day)

Today's Notes (Highlights, Thoughts, Feelings, What Could You Improve On?)

"Fructose (the sugar found in fruits) is kind to the pancreas and its absorption into the body uses minimal energy."

Today's Date:

Morning
(work towards continuing your night time dry fast up until at least 12pm)

Afternoon
(get hydrating with fresh fruit or even better slow juiced fruits/berries/melons)

Evening
(aim to wind down to a dry fast by around 6pm to 7pm)

Night
(work your way up to dry fasting from the evening until 12pm the following day)

Today's Notes (Highlights, Thoughts, Feelings, What Could You Improve On?)

"Fruits have the highest healing energy frequencies among all food groups. Vegetables are the next highest. Cooked meats rank the lowest."

Today's Date:

Morning
(work towards continuing your night time dry fast up until at least 12pm)

Afternoon
(get hydrating with fresh fruit or even better slow juiced fruits/berries/melons)

Evening
(aim to wind down to a dry fast by around 6pm to 7pm)

Night
(work your way up to dry fasting from the evening until 12pm the following day)

Today's Notes (Highlights, Thoughts, Feelings, What Could You Improve On?)

"Mucus congestion (caused by dairy products) leads to a lack of mineral utilization (Calcium, Magnesium, Potassium, etc)."

Today's Date:

Morning
(work towards continuing your night time dry fast up until at least 12pm)

Afternoon
(get hydrating with fresh fruit or even better slow juiced fruits/berries/melons)

Evening
(aim to wind down to a dry fast by around 6pm to 7pm)

Night
(work your way up to dry fasting from the evening until 12pm the following day)

Today's Notes (Highlights, Thoughts, Feelings, What Could You Improve On?)

"Did you know that fruit juice (slow juiced) will offer you more Calcium than Cow's Milk?"

Today's Date:

──────────────── **Morning** ────────────────

(work towards continuing your night time dry fast up until at least 12pm)

──────────────── **Afternoon** ────────────────

(get hydrating with fresh fruit or even better slow juiced fruits/berries/melons)

──────────────── **Evening** ────────────────

(aim to wind down to a dry fast by around 6pm to 7pm)

──────────────── **Night** ────────────────

(work your way up to dry fasting from the evening until 12pm the following day)

Today's Notes (Highlights, Thoughts, Feelings, What Could You Improve On?)

"Your body will use sweating (fevers), vomiting, diarrhea, frequent urination, colds, flus, and daily elimination as means to detox a toxic state. Let it run its course."

Today's Date:

―――――――――――― **Morning** ――――――――――――
(work towards continuing your night time dry fast up until at least 12pm)

―――――――――――― **Afternoon** ――――――――――――
(get hydrating with fresh fruit or even better slow juiced fruits/berries/melons)

―――――――――――― **Evening** ――――――――――――
(aim to wind down to a dry fast by around 6pm to 7pm)

―――――――――――― **Night** ――――――――――――
(work your way up to dry fasting from the evening until 12pm the following day)

Today's Notes (Highlights, Thoughts, Feelings, What Could You Improve On?)

"Pain is merely a sign of energy blockage(s) resulting from acidosis. Alkalization is the key (through detoxification)."

Today's Date:

Morning

(work towards continuing your night time dry fast up until at least 12pm)

Afternoon

(get hydrating with fresh fruit or even better slow juiced fruits/berries/melons)

Evening

(aim to wind down to a dry fast by around 6pm to 7pm)

Night

(work your way up to dry fasting from the evening until 12pm the following day)

Today's Notes (Highlights, Thoughts, Feelings, What Could You Improve On?)

"Keep on loving! Love is alkalizing, it improves digestion and kidney elimination. Your blood and lymph flow will also improve."

Today's Date:

———————————— Morning ————————————
(work towards continuing your night time dry fast up until at least 12pm)

———————————— Afternoon ————————————
(get hydrating with fresh fruit or even better slow juiced fruits/berries/melons)

———————————— Evening ————————————
(aim to wind down to a dry fast by around 6pm to 7pm)

———————————— Night ————————————
(work your way up to dry fasting from the evening until 12pm the following day)

Today's Notes (Highlights, Thoughts, Feelings, What Could You Improve On?)

"Ensure any amalgam fillings in your teeth are replaced with composite fillings – preferably by a holistic dentist."

Today's Date:

Morning
(work towards continuing your night time dry fast up until at least 12pm)

Afternoon
(get hydrating with fresh fruit or even better slow juiced fruits/berries/melons)

Evening
(aim to wind down to a dry fast by around 6pm to 7pm)

Night
(work your way up to dry fasting from the evening until 12pm the following day)

Today's Notes (Highlights, Thoughts, Feelings, What Could You Improve On?)

"Use parsley to detox mercury out of your body."

Today's Date:

———— Morning ————
(work towards continuing your night time dry fast up until at least 12pm)

———— Afternoon ————
(get hydrating with fresh fruit or even better slow juiced fruits/berries/melons)

———— Evening ————
(aim to wind down to a dry fast by around 6pm to 7pm)

———— Night ————
(work your way up to dry fasting from the evening until 12pm the following day)

Today's Notes (Highlights, Thoughts, Feelings, What Could You Improve On?)

"Sleep is very vital for your healing. Wind down by 7pm and aim to be in bed by 10pm to 10:30pm (if possible)."

Today's Date:

―――――――――――― **Morning** ――――――――――――

(work towards continuing your night time dry fast up until at least 12pm)

―――――――――――― **Afternoon** ――――――――――――

(get hydrating with fresh fruit or even better slow juiced fruits/berries/melons)

―――――――――――― **Evening** ――――――――――――

(aim to wind down to a dry fast by around 6pm to 7pm)

―――――――――――― **Night** ――――――――――――

(work your way up to dry fasting from the evening until 12pm the following day)

Today's Notes (Highlights, Thoughts, Feelings, What Could You Improve On?)

"Keep a positive mindset. Remind yourself that everything is possible & you WILL achieve your goals"

CPSIA information can be obtained
at www.ICGtesting.com
Printed in the USA
LVHW081307130619
621113LV00018B/503/P